Herbalist's Guide
to
Preventing the Common Cold

Janet Partlow

August 2014

The Herbalist's Guide to Preventing the Common Cold

It was nearly forty years ago that I became a physician assistant (PA). A PA works in modern medicine, side by side with doctors to diagnose and treat common illnesses. More complicated health issues are managed by the doctors. As a PA over these years, I had many opportunities to help people deal with the common cold. And as a PA, I shared the common complaint of many of my clients: *"We can put people on the moon. Why can't we put a stop to the common cold?"*

In my last years of working as a PA, I worked in a college health clinic. It was incredibly frustrating to me when a student would come in, asking me to help her prevent catching the cold that was currently rampaging through the dorm. I would trot out the usual modern medicine suggestions of washing her hands, getting plenty of sleep, yada, yada, yada but both she and I had a sense of futility, knowing how unlikely it was that those approaches would really do the trick. Indeed, I would watch waves of viruses sweep through the campus, sucking energy, time and health from students who really needed to be at the top of their game. As a healer, I felt helpless.

When I began learning herbal medicine almost twenty years ago, it was like a miracle to find out that the ancient herbal traditions had in fact a number of medicinal plants they used to prevent and/or treat the common cold. These herbs have not been evaluated by the FDA for efficacy (see the foreword on FDA precautions). However the people of China, India and ancient Europe have used these remedies for thousands of years and have a long experience that tells them that these herbs can work.

So one of the first things my earliest herbal instructor KP Khalsa taught us was what he called the viral raid. Though I was interested and eager to begin my herbal training, I was quite skeptical that herbs could actually work against a cold. In my modern medicine training I felt we were pretty much brainwashed to believe that all herbs were useless, sold by snake oil salesmen, a waste of time and money and dangerous to boot. But since modern medicine never had offered anything really helpful against cold viruses, it seemed worth a trial. So I thought I'd start by trying these herbs on myself.

At that time I was working in the college, exposed to the viruses running through that community. I had developed an autoimmune disease (rheumatoid arthritis) about a few year previously, so I was particularly vulnerable to catching these viruses. In my days in this clinic, I generally got about 6-10 viral illnesses a year. They would course through my system for the standard 7 - 10 days. I'd be miserable from the cold and after my immune system woke up and kicked it out, the arthritis would flare up for a couple of weeks and I would have a lot of joint pain. As a result, I was very motivated to find a way to shut down these colds.

So I started experimenting with KP Khalsa's viral raid. Over the next year or so I figured out what worked best for me and began to utilize it. I then shared it with family and friends, who were very excited to report back as to how well it worked. Finally I began sharing it with patients; they too got excellent results.

Today I get maybe one viral illness a year. A few times a year viruses will make a sneak attempt on me, but I know what to look for and I know how to stop them. I have a large group of family, friends & clients who also use the viral raid and swear by it.

So in this book, I will share these suggestions. I suggest you try them out for yourself and see what works. Each of us is different, so what works for me may not work for you. But I will suggest a number of different approaches you can try and I feel confident that at least one of these will work for you. Really, what do you have to lose?

Some Herbal Precautions

In this book on herbal remedies there are several suggestions for herbs you might want to try. These herbs have not been evaluated by the Food & Drug Administration for effectiveness or safety. When you buy bottles of prepared herbs, the FDA requires this statement on the label.

In addition, herbalists are not licensed to diagnosis, treat or cure any disease.

In general it is recommended that if you have any questions about these herbal products, consult your physician.

Now this is good information, as far as it goes. It's also important to understand that few if any medical practitioners get much training in herbal medicine. So if you take your plant questions to them, they may not be able to offer any help. Pharmacists are also not generally well-trained in herbal medicine, so that is a challenge as well. A good option is to see a naturopathic physician, who is trained both in modern medicine and herbal medicine. Some naturopaths have a stronger background in herbs so ask around to find one in your community who can help you.

A general rule that I follow in making herbal suggestions is that if you are taking several medications for significant health issues, it is best not to blend herbs with those medications unless you have consulted with a practitioner who knows both herbs and your medications. Again, your best bet here is a naturopath.

In the back of this book is a resource section. It has specific notes on how to find other healers such as herbalists, naturopaths, acupuncturists and more. Check it out!

The Viral Raid

Here's how it works:

• First you have to start to pay attention to how a cold virus typically shows up for you. It's different for each person, but each of us tends to have our own warning signs. For example, I notice in the earliest days of a virus, my sinuses inexplicably start to run and I tend to have a runny nose, with clear mucous. Along with this I get what I call the snorts (post-nasal drainage) that just won't stop. My throat gets itchy and scratchy. I may have sneezing. I may also have some aches and pains; often these show up in places that tend to be sore. For example, if you have recurrent problems with a sore neck, you may have a recurrence of neck pain. This can be an early virus warning sign

My husband has the three sneeze rule. He will unleash a volley of sneezes, which are not uncommon for him because he also has the occasional seasonal allergies. But if he has more than three sneezes in a row, he and I look at each other and go "*Uh oh. Time for a viral raid.*"

These symptoms are typical of a cold virus in its earliest stages and in fact make sense in light of the way the virus finds its way into your system. Typically a virus enters by falling on a moist mucous membrane surface; your eyes, your nose, your mouth and your throat. Once on this surface, the virus enters the cells and starts to replicate itself. This is particularly true in the throat.

• Once you notice these symptoms, it's time to take action. In the first 24 hours of a cold virus, you can usually shut it down. But you have to be paying attention so as to know to take action. Here's what you do:

<u>You need to have these things on hand:</u>

• Zinc lozenges. Zinc has been proven to block the replication of viruses in the mucous membranes. The trick is that you have to apply the zinc where the viruses are, which is why you use lozenges.

There are many brands of zinc lozenges out there, and a lot of them taste really horrid. So I looked around and did the research for you. I prefer Zand lozenges. They work, they taste good and the price is right. There is one called elderberry zinc and another called echinacea zinc, both of which I recommend. I keep a bag of these in the house and in that 24 hour window, I slowly suck on 8-10 of these lozenges. This helps stop the virus at the front door.

Amazon.com sells these, though many supplement/vitamin stores do so as well. You can google Amazon for Zand brand zinc lozenges to learn more.

• Vitamin C: In the KP Khalsa viral raid, Vitamin C plays a key role, so I take it. He recommended about 2000 milligrams all at once. There are many sources of vitamin C out there; one of my favorite is the Emerg-C packets, easily available in supplement stores or online. Again, you can google Amazon.com and check out their Emerg-C, including what people say about it.

Now we move on to the herbs:
• Astragalus (*Astragalus propinquus*) : This is an herb that is native to China and has been used in Traditional Chinese Medicine for thousands of years. It is believed to be an herb that supports the immune system as it does its job; in doing so, it helps your immune system chase out the viruses. KP Khalsa talked about how it makes the bone marrow more active in building the white cells that fight viruses, as well as increasing the release of antibodies.

Michael Tierra describes it as an adaptogen herb, which is a type of medicinal plant which increases energy and builds resistance to weakness and disease. In Chinese medicine they think of astragalus as a master Qi replenisher and a guardian of the immune system.

We use the root. Traditionally it was put into soup and the soup was then eaten. There are other ways to take it. Here are the usual doses:
To shut down a virus in the first 24 hours:
=Take 15- 20 capsules of powdered root **OR**
=Take 4-5 full droppers of Astragalus tincture. Herb Pharm makes an excellent tincture that is widely available.   **OR**

=Take 5 teaspoons of powdered astragalus and add a couple of cups of water. Bring to a boil and let simmer at a low temperature for 30 minutes. Then drink it up. As herbs go, it has a mild, bland taste.

Check the back of the book for the page on how to herbal recipes. This will give you the basics you need to make decisions about which form of herb to use and where to find it.

You can google Horizon herbs and use their search link to find pictures of herbs along with information about the plants. Horizon also sells live plants you can put in your own garden.

Preventative Maintenance Against Cold Viruses

So this is the viral raid: what you do in the first 24 hours to shut down a cold virus. In my personal and professional experience, this works about 90% of the time to shut down a virus.

\tNow we move on to the medicinal herbs that can be used preventatives. These are herbs you take on a daily basis for several months to stop a cold virus before it gets a foothold.

I recommend that you start preventatives in September and take them throughout the cold season, which in our area (Pacific NW) runs into April/May. I usually take the summer off from preventatives, relying instead on good sleep and good self care to get me through. If I do run across a summer cold, then I will jump on the viral raid treatment.

• Black Elderberry *(Sambucus nigra or canadensis)* This is an herb that grows in Europe and eastern North America. Our ancestors from the British Isles and Ireland used it extensively in the fall and winter to prevent viral illnesses. It is believed to open up the pores to bring out heat and fluids, thus reducing a fever. It is said to open up the lungs and helps in bringing up mucous. Some recent research work in Europe found that two chemicals in elderberry can prevent the flu viruses from invading throat cells.

It is also a bitter herb, which means it helps stimulate the liver to produce more bile and to clean itself out. This is important in viral illnesses because the liver is like your own personal garbage person: it clears out the viral garbage and carts it away. You know what happens if there is a strike and household garbage starts to build up along your street? Well, the same sort of thing can occur in your body. A healthy liver that is moving out toxins & viruses means that you are less likely to get sick.

We use the berries. These are made into a syrup. A commercial preparation called Sambucol can be readily purchased in herb and supplement stores. It is also available through Amazon. (I often recommend Amazon because the price is very good and you can also read the reviews of other people who tried it.)

You can also make your own syrup and keep it in the refrigerator. I start in September and take 1 tablespoon a day (for adults). It is safe for children 3 years and up, but adjust the dose: ½ to 1 tsp a day.

Check the back of the book for the recipe for homemade elderberry syrup.

Precautions: if you make your own syrup, be sure to find black elderberries. In the Pacific Northwest there are red elderberries, but they can be toxic to eat. There are also blue elderberries and the jury is still out on whether these can also be toxic. The safest thing is to use only black elderberries. Check the resource page in the back of the book for places to get herbs.

• Medicinal Mushrooms. I live in the wet side of the Pacific Northwest which is mushroom heaven. Mushrooms of many sorts erupt all around us, especially in the fall. In the last few years I became very interested in this bounty and have spent a great deal of time learning whatever I could find about them, especially medicinal mushrooms.

I used to think that medicinal mushrooms were like herbs in that you need a different species for different problems. When it comes to colds, that does not appear to be true. Many kinds of these fungi are phenomenally effective at building up the immune system.. So you can take them on a daily basis through the cold season and they will keep your immune system strong. One PA friend of mine started doing this a few years ago and has noticed a dramatic decrease in her viral illnesses, despite the fact that she works full time in a family practice clinic, where she gets exposed to every virus on the planet.

Some mushrooms which I think are best at building up the immune system include:
• Reishi
• Turkey Tail

- Shitake
- Cordyceps
- Agarikon

So how do you go about getting medicinal mushrooms in your body? There are a couple of excellent choices.

Paul Stamets of Fungi Perfecti has developed a great mushroom blend which he calls Host Defense: My Community. It has 17 different mushrooms blended together, to work synergistically to keep the immune system strong. It comes in capsule form and you take 2 capsules a day throughout the September to May cold season. Google Fungi Perfecti to find their website.

I also like to work with the people of Mushroom Harvest in Ohio. They sell bulk mushroom powders: one is a 5 mushroom blend and another is a 14 mushroom blend. You can buy anywhere from 4 ounces to a pound of these blends. You take 1-2 tsps a day. You can make up your own capsules (see the back of this ebook for instructions on how to do this). If you use their blend, you need 4 - 8 capsules a day.

Or you can simply stir the powder into a couple of cups of hot water, let it sit for a few minutes and drink. You can also add these powders to soups.

I like Mushroom Harvest because not only do they really know their mushrooms, but they offer them at a reasonable price. Google Mushroom Harvest to find their website.

- A word about echinacea: many people use echinacea to shut down an early cold. If this is what you use and it works for you, by all means stick with it. Above all, good healers believe that you need to stick with what works for you.

I don't use echinacea. It doesn't seem to work for me. In addition, there are some suggestions that for people with autoimmune disease, it may fire up the overactive parts of the immune system even more than usual. So for me it's not a good choice.

It is an herb native to a fairly limited range in the North American prairies, but it has been extensively over harvested, so this is another reason I don't recommend it. The demand for it has not only caused over harvesting, but also raised the cost, so these are other factors.

Finally, Michael Tierra who is one of America's top herbalists, speaks of it as a cold damp herb; Generally the cold virus is also a cold and damp condition: does it make sense to chase a cold virus with a cold & damp herb? I don't think so. In contrast, astragalus is slightly warming, so it is a much better fit. It literally grows like a weed wherever it is planted, so the risk of over harvesting is low. Its cost is low. So for me, there are better choices. Let's keep echinacea around for the times we might really need it.

Some non-herbal approaches to immune support

There are a number of strategies we can use to keep our immune systems healthy besides plants. From the world of the herbalist, these are some of my favorites.

Get to bed by 11 pm each night and get the hours of sleep that your body needs. My understanding of this comes from Traditional Chinese Medicine (TCM). In that world of healing, they believe in a 24 hour body clock, whereby every two hours one organ system is at its most effective and powerful. The time from 11 pm to 3 am is the time of the gallbladder and liver. Earlier I wrote about how the liver takes out the viral garbage. It turns out if you are asleep during this time you are giving the liver its best help for fighting this cold. Some people are naturally night owls and find it hard to be asleep by 11 pm. In that case, just lie down and rest. That works almost as well

Limit your intake of sugar: sugar is documented to suppress the immune system. Since we are trying to get the immune system at its best to fight the virus, sugar is counter-productive. By sugar I mean cane sugar. Honey in small amounts is fine.

Wash hands & cover coughs. This is the usual advice from modern medicine and it's good advice. I wrote earlier about how virus particles enter our bodies through contact with a moist mucous membrane. Sometimes we get the virus on our hands, then rub our eyes. This is one sure-fire way to get exposed. So hand-washing is very useful.

In the world of the herbalist, one of the greatest enemies I see in all my clients is stress. Stress plays a key role in knocking back the immune system. From my years as a healer, it is clear that most adults have heavy stress and some have extraordinary stress. It seems to be a chronic issue in all our lives.

We don't always have a choice about some of that stress, but we do have a choice about how we manage it. It is beyond the scope of this book to go over this topic in detail, but briefly, here are some of my favorite tools to manage stress. See if any of these speak to you:

Some sort of meditation practice. You can find classes on Mindfulness Meditation at community centers and colleges. Yoga studios often teach meditation as well as Buddhist temples.

Yoga: this combines breathing exercise, movement/stretching and meditation. A three for one deal! Check for local Yoga classes and studios. Community centers and community colleges often have evening classes.

Qi Gong – This is a TCM movement practice. Acupuncturists are often required to take these classes throughout their training and afterwards, many of them teach Qi Gong. Try and find an acupuncturist in your community who can teach this. I have found this to be wonderfully relaxing. Tai Qi is a martial arts form of Qi Gong and some people prefer to do this.

Breathing exercises. Andrew Weil has a wonderful CD called <u>Breathing: The Master Key to Self Healing</u>. It has eight exercises which can be remarkably helpful in clearing the effects of chronic stress. I especially like the 4/7/8 breath for its powerful ability to calm people down. You can google 4/7/8 breath on the internet and download this for free.

Guided Imagery for Relieving Stress: Bellaruth Naperstak is a therapist who started a company called Health Journeys. She uses guided visualizations for a wide variety of health issues. Her CD on Relieving Stress is excellent and is one of my personal key tools for stress management. Google <u>healthjourneys.com</u> to find her website.

Regular exercise: walking, running, strength training, flexibility training. This plays an important role in keeping our circulatory, lymph & liver systems strong to flush out those viruses and also to clear out the biochemical effects of stress.

When the Viral Raid Fails

There are times where despite my best efforts, the viral raid fails and I end up with a cold. That happened this summer: I got my first cold in over a year.

There were some reasons for this. Basically I got sloppy in my self-care habits. It was summer, so I was staying up later than usual, enjoying the warm summer nights. I was eating lots of ice cream (think of all the sugar in that ice cream, inhibiting my immune system). I go to an exercise class at the gym three times a week where I use the gym's equipment. I'd gotten careless about washing my hands afterwards.   All these things conspired against me and I got a cold. The herbal viral raid failed.

But I wasn't upset. I believe it is important to have the occasional cold: I think the immune system and defenses of the respiratory system need an occasional reminder about the enemy. So I moved on to the final part of the herbal remedies for treating colds. This is what I did.

• I continued to take astragalus, 5 capsules a day. This provides good immune support to the body as it works to clear the virus.
• I had some medicinal mushroom blend for immune defense, so I took a couple of teaspoons a day. Once again I was focusing on supporting my immune system.
• I canceled my clients for a couple of days to stay home and take care of myself. Several of them expressed real appreciation that I had not exposed them to this summer cold. I was surprised and grateful at their support. It's a good reminder that none of us are indispensable and it's okay to stay home and take care of ourselves.
• I made a point of resting, taking naps when I felt like it, and going to bed early. This was a huge help.
• I sent my husband out to get me some chicken soup from the local Asian Deli. It's full of veggies, tofu and chicken. I'm a firm believer in the healing properties of chicken soup.

Doing all these things, the virus cleared within 48 hours. So even though the viral raid failed, I used herbs & good self-care to shorten the course of this cold.

Other respiratory/immune herbs to consider:
- Boneset for aches & pains and fever. This is a very bitter tasting herb, so capsules are best. 5 capsules a day.
- Yerba Santa is a decent herb for congestion. I have not had great luck finding herbs to clear congestion, but this is the best of the bunch. Tincture works well here: 30 drops (one dropper full) three times a day as needed.
- Essential oil steams: I like to use Eucalyptus, Rosemary and/or Thyme essential oils in a steam. Get a pot of water boiling and pour it into a heavy glass bowl. Let it cool to a comfortable steam level. Put in 1-2 drops of each oil (these are potent herbs and less is best!) Get a heavy towel and drape over your head and the bowl. Breathe in the steam for 10 - 15 minutes. This can have several uses:
- The oils help open the sinuses and lungs and promote decongestion.
- All of them have antimicrobial and antiviral effects; by getting them deep into sinuses and lungs you can often chase out the viruses.

Herbal Recipes

There are many ways to make herbal preparations and each herbalist has her/his favorites. You need to decide what works for you. In this book I'm writing down my recipes. These are simple, basic and can be easily done in your own home kitchen.

A great reference book for making herbal preparations is: The <u>Herbal Medicine Maker's Handbook</u> by James Green. This book has everything you'd ever want to know about herbal recipes and is the place I go when I am stuck.

<u>Tinctures</u> Herbs are often sold in tincture form. A commercially prepared tincture has some sort of alcohol (usually pure grain alcohol); the plant material soaks in the alcohol for a while during which time the alcohol acts as a solvent and extracts all the medicine from the plant. The plant material is then strained off and you are left with the medicinal tincture.

Advantages of tinctures are these:
- They last a long time, if stored in a dark bottle in a cool dry place.
- They are easy and convenient to find in stores, and to take.
- They may be better absorbed by the body, especially if you have digestive issues.
- The medicine is very quickly available to the body.

Disadvantages that I see are:
- They are alcohol based so for people with alcoholism issues, they are not a great idea.
- They can be expensive, because you pay for not only the plants but also the alcohol solvent. For example if you want to take a month's worth of feverfew for headache prevention, the commercial cost of that tincture will run about $80.00. So it's something to consider.
- Some people really dislike the taste of the herbs in tincture, which means they may not consistently use the medicine.

Here's the "folk method" for making tinctures

- Get some dried plant material from the store. Or collect the material from your garden, lay out in a single layer on a window screen type of material so air can circulate. Leave in a cool, dry place until the plants are well dried. Another method is to bundle up the herbs at the base, and hang the bundle flower tips down so all the good medicine runs into the leaves and is dried there.
- Take a clean jar with a good tight lid. Take your plant material and crumble or use a food processor to chop it down to bits and fill the jar 2/3 - 3/4 full of dried herb.
- Pour an alcohol solvent over it. I use potato-based vodka 100 proof, which is gluten free and cheap. Pour the vodka over the plant material nearly to the top of the jar, leaving about 1 inch space. Stir around to get the plant material well soaked. Cap off tightly with a clean lid.
- Put your jar in a sunny window, in a place where you will see it daily. Shake it down daily to stir the herbs and alcohol together. As the days progress, you will notice the alcohol is taking on the color of the plants, and the plant material is becoming brittle and lifeless.
- After 2 weeks, your tincture is done. Get another clean jar and a funnel. Line the funnel with cheesecloth and strain off your tincture. When most of the liquid seems drained off, bundle up the cheesecloth and squeeze hard, draining off the last bits.
- Cap off your jar of tincture tightly. Label and date. It's best to use a dark bottle, but the poor man's alternative is to use a mason jar and just put the tincture in a brown paper bag. Store in a cool, dark place.

Powdered herbs When I work with a client who has decided to try some herbs, we need to sort out what is the best way for him to take them. Some people are fine with tinctures: they like the ease of purchase. Other people (like me) struggle with the intense taste of some medicinal herbs, so for folks like me, powdered herbs in capsule form work best.

Advantages of powdered capsules:
- Definitely cheaper, especially if you make your own,

- You can avoid the taste of the herbs. Some herbalists consider this is a disadvantage, because the taste of the herb can have its own medicinal effects. But I tend to be practical about it: we have to find a way to get the medicine down and capsules will bypass the yuck factor.

Disadvantages of powdered capsules
- Some people have trouble swallowing capsules
- Powdered herbs tend to lose their quality quickly. I recommend using them within 6 months of purchase. There are also a lot of bad quality herb capsules being sold out there, so only buy capsules from an herb store or supplement store you trust.
- They involve more work if you go with making your own capsules.

How to make your own powdered capsules
- Get some dried plant material from the store. Or collect the material from your garden, lay out in a   single layer on a window screen type of material so air can circulate. Leave in a cool, dry place until the plants are well dried. Another method is to bundle up the herbs at the base, and hang the bundle flower tips down so all the good medicine runs into the leaves and is dried there.
- Take your plant material and crumble it down. Then use a coffee mill or a food processor and grind it down to a fine powder. Some root herbs are hard to grind and may destroy your machine, so test a small amount first. One strategy with fibrous or tough roots is to freeze them for a few hours, then grind. The freezing makes them brittle and thus easier to work with. Some roots are really tough, so it's just easier to buy from the company which has already ground them down for you. (See herbal resources page.)
- The best way I have found to capsule herbs is to buy The Capsule Machine for "00" size capsules. This machine is available online or from your local herb/supplement store. You also need some size "00" capsules; I buy these online through Amazon because they are cheaper. Follow the instructions that come with the machine. These capsule machines produce 24 caps at a pop and are really slick. At

our house, we sit and make capsules while we watch movies. It works well.

Herbal teas - Let's say you want to make an herbal tea to chase out the cold symptoms. Here's a possible suggestion: Mix 1 teaspoon of dried yarrow leaves & flowers, plus 1 tsp. peppermint leaves in a large cup. Pour 2 cups boiling water over these herbs and let them sit for 10 - 15 minutes. Now strain out the tea leaves and drink.

This is a medicinal tea so it will be strong. It may not taste great, but that's because you need to take enough herbs to get the effects you want. You can make it more palatable by adding honey.

Here's another favorite tea I use when I have a nasty full-on cold; I call it my virus chaser. I use fresh kitchen herbs. Get a saucepan and put in:
• One thumb size piece of fresh ginger, peeled and chopped into bits.
• 2 cloves of fresh garlic, peeled and chopped into bits.
• Squeeze out the juice of one lemon. You can also peel off the yellow part and add to the tea. All this chopping can be done by hand or quite easily in a food processor.

Now add 3 cups of water to the saucepan and bring the mixture to a boil. Reduce to a very low simmer and let it steep for 30 minutes. Now strain out the herbs and add honey to taste. Once again, it doesn't taste great but it is very effective in chasing away the worst of a cold virus.

Infused herbal oil for topical use: I really like to made infused herbal oils and I use them for all kinds of health issues. These are kitchen/ food herbs which you soak in oil, either over the stove or in a jar in a window. After the oil is finished, you strain off the herbs, label, date and store in the refrigerator to be applied topically as needed. Here is a good recipe for an herbal chest rub, similar to the Vicks we all remember from childhood.
• Get a handful of fresh eucalyptus leaves, a handful of rosemary leaves, a handful of thyme leaves and a handful of peppermint leaves. With fresh herbs you lay them out on a window screen

overnight to evaporate off some of their moisture; this prevents the later formation of mold on your infused oil. You can also buy dried herbs, which eliminates the window screen step.

- Put your dried herbs in a double boiler pan. The bottom pan has a few inches of water while the herbs go inside the inner pan. Cover the herbs with oil so that it's about 1 inch above the plants. I'm a kitchen herbalist so I like to use olive oil. Other people buy almond, grape seed or jojoba oil: your choice.

- Bring the water in the lower pan to the lowest possible simmer. Put the lid on the pan of oil/herbs and let the mixture slowly cook away on the stove over several hours. As the water evaporates from the herbs, it will condense on the pan lid. Take a clean towel and periodically mop out this liquid so it doesn't fall back into the oil. This process takes about six hours so do it on a day when you plan to be in the house. When done, let the mixture cool so you can safely handle it.

- Take your finished oil/flower product and strain it through cheesecloth or paper towels. Let it drain fully, and squeeze every last bit of goodness out of the plant mass. Strain into clean jars; put on a tight lid, labeling and dating your oil. You should be able to smell the herbs in the oil. If you wish you can add a couple of drops each of essential oils of eucalyptus, rosemary, thyme and peppermint: these boost the smell and may also make it more effective as a chest rub for tight, congested lungs.

Elderberry Honey Recipe

Herbal honey is a traditional way to preserve herbal medicines over time, and also a tasty way to get things down (this is especially true for picky eaters like kids). Since this was a traditional family syrup, there are many different ways to prepare it.

In this recipe we are making elderberry honey as a fall/winter virus preventative. Generally the easiest way to get the berries is to buy black elderberries from a reputable herb source (see the resource list in the back of this book.

You can buy the berries whole or ground up. If they are whole, run them through an herb mill or food processor to reduce them to a powder. Then put the herbs in a double boiler pan: the bottom pan needs a few inches of water and the top pan holds the herbs. Cover the elderberries with honey to about 1 inch above the level of the herbs. Stir to make sure all the herbs are well-coated. Put a lid on the double boiler pan and bring it to a simmer. Then reduce the stove top heat to the lowest possible setting and let the herbs and honey infuse. Plan on doing this for about 4-6 hours.

Check the mixture occasionally. As you lift the lid of the pan, you will notice moisture has condensed on the lid. Use a clean towel to mop this out. Repeat several times over the hours the mixture is infusing; this process also helps remove excess moisture.

Taste the honey sporadically. When the honey picks up the taste of the herbs, you can take it off the stove. Pour the mixture through a fine mesh metal sieve to remove the herbs; pour the honey into a clean jar, put on a lid, and label and date. I store elderberry honey in the refrigerator.

Some people add other ingredients: grated fresh ginger, cloves, or cinnamon for taste.

Sage Honey Recipe for treating a cold

Kitchen sage is an herb that many traditional cultures considered sacred. They believed it had great powers to heal many ailments. In fact, the plant's genus name, Salvia, means "to save".

Cultures around the world have infused sage in honey for preserving it and increasing the medicinal properties for many symptoms such as headaches, sore throats, tonsillitis, insomnia, colds and flu, stomach distress and all of the respiratory ailments. Sage soothes the nerves too.

Raw honey also has medicinal properties just by itself. It is antibacterial and fights off the colds and flu. It boosts your immune system so it can do its job of fighting off viruses. When sage is infused in the honey you get a powerful herbal remedy that will aid you in recovering from colds and flu.

Sage is rich in calcium, magnesium, potassium and zinc. These minerals are used up when your body is fighting off viruses. Sage is also rich in essential fatty acids and vitamin C.

To make sage herbal honey, pick unblemished leaves and tear into small pieces. Fill a small glass canning jar with the leaves and pour raw honey over the leaves. Stir with the end of a wooden spoon until all the leaves are soaked with the honey. Add more honey to fill the jar and cap tightly. Set the honey on your counter and stir it every day for 2-6 weeks. You can also just turn the jar over each day and let the honey bubble up through the leaves to keep it all soaked. You can use the honey within a day or so, but the longer it sets, the more medicinal properties are pulled out of the leaves and into the honey. You can leave the leaves in or strain them out.

To use your sage herbal honey for sore throats, just swallow a teaspoonful several times a day and let the honey set on the throat and soothe it. Or you can put 1 tablespoon of the honey in a cup and pour boiling water over it to make a tea.

Herbal Resources

There are many places all over the world to buy herbs. I live in the Pacific Northwest and I believe it is very important to use plants that are mostly grown in my own bioregion, so I choose local herb sellers. I encourage you to do the same.

If you live someplace far away from the Northwest, I encourage you to check out your local herb stores, herbalists and supplement stores to find out about what herb sellers are available in your area. Check out your local farmer's markets : this is often a good place to find herbs.

One of my favorite strategies is to google "Herbs in_____anytown, USA" and see what comes up. This can help lead you to sources of herbs.

Try and find good products. Stay away from the big box stores. You can certainly buy cheap herbs at Walmart but I promise you, their primary interest is in making money. You want to spend your hard-earned money on powerful & healthy herbs that will actually give you the results you are looking for.

Places to buy herb products:
- Mountain Rose in Eugene, Oregon Use google to find them on the internet
- Herb Pharm in Williams, Oregon A great resource for tinctured herbs. Use google to find them.
- Mushroom Harvest in Athen, Ohio Use google to find them on the internet
- Fungi Perfecti near Olympia, Washington. Use google to find them on the internet.
- Western Herb Products in Gold Bar, Washington They are not on the internet, so you need to contact through their phone (360) 793-1033.

A wonderful resource for buying herb plants. They do a great job of shipping live plants:

• Horizon Herbs in Williams, Oregon. Use google to find them on the internet. You can also find live herb plants at your local farmer's market and some local nurseries.

My Favorite Herbal Reference Books

    My first herbal instructor told us to be sure to have a big bookshelf because we would be collecting lots of herbal references. I didn't believe him. He was right; my office today has a huge shelf of books. Here is a short list of some of my favorites.

Herbal Defense	Robin Landis & KP Khalsa
Home Medicine Chest	Rosemary Gladstar
Rosemary Gladstar's Family Herbal	Rosemary Gladstar
The Holistic Herbal	David Hoffman
The Herbalist's Way	Nancy Phillips
Medicinal Plants of the Pacific West	Michael Moore
Medicinal Plants of the Mountain West	Michael Moore
The Herbal Medicine Maker's Handbook	James Green
The Way of Ayurvedic Herbs	KP Khalsa and Michael Tierra
The Way of Chinese Herbs	Michael Tierra
Herbal Therapy & Supplements	Merrily Kuhn and David Winston
The Earthwise Herbal	Matthew Wood
The Rainforest Home Remedies	Rosita Arvigo & Nadine Epstein
Healing Herbs in Ireland	Paula O'Regan
Plant Spirit Medicine 2nd Edition	Eliot Cowan
Medicinal Mushrooms	Christopher Hobbs

Other resources:

When we are working to improve our health, I believe that we all need a village of healers. Besides having a solid primary care physician, you may also want to consider these alternative medicine healers:

Herbalists There are local herbalists, some of whom are members of indigenous tribes or have other family traditions in which they have been trained. You need to ask around to find these people since some of them do not advertise. Local herb or supplement stores can often help you here.

You can also google the American Herbalist Guild. This is a professional organization that provides a certification for herbalists who choose to seek a professional credential. Look under "Our Members" and you will find a search mode for locating AHG herbalists in your area.

Naturopathic Physicians These are medical doctors, trained in modern medicine and also in alternative medicine. You can google the American Association of Naturopathic Physicians which has a search mode by which you can find such doctors in your community.

Acupuncturists Acupuncturists are formally trained and licensed in Traditional Chinese Medicine and/or Five Element Classic Chinese Medicine. You can find one in your area by asking around, or google the National Certification Commission for Acupuncture and Oriental Medicine. They have a search engine so you can find an acupuncturist in your area.

Healing Touch practitioners Healing Touch is an energy healing modality which works to bring the human energy field (chakras & aura) back into balance. My first training in energy medicine in 1995 was Healing Touch; I continue to use it today on myself and my clients because it is truly a profound healing modality. There are certified HT practitioners who have completed the full training (five levels). You can google Healing Touch International and check their directory for certified practitioners in your area.

<u>Eden Energy Medicine practitioners</u> Donna Eden is a phenomenal energy medicine healer who over the last 45 years developed her own energy medicine healing tools and training program for healers. This is yet another phenomenal energy healing modality that I use on myself and clients. You can google Donna Eden at Innersource to find her state by state directory of certified Eden Energy Medicine practitioners.

My background as an herbalist

I grew up in a family of healers. My grandma was a nurse and my mom studied nursing during World War II. My great-grandfather HW Partlow became a doctor in 1885 in Michigan and continued his medical practice when he came to Olympia, Washington where I now live. Several of his descendants became physicians. There was a certain pressure on me to become a doctor but somehow the pressure never quite took. I ended up finishing my college degree by becoming a physician assistant (PA) with a specialty in women's health care. I later went back to the University of Washington where I got additional training in Medex NW, becoming a PA in family medicine in 1980. I took an early retirement from that work in 2002.

Around 1995 the medicine of plants began to call to me. I had developed rheumatoid arthritis and despite the efforts of an excellent rheumatologist, nothing she did or prescribed offered any relief. I was also working in a college health center; many of my young adult patients were very interested in herbal medicine and were disappointed that I had no training and expertise to offer in this area. I was desperate to find relief from my arthritis pain and also under pressure from my patients, so I began my studies in herbal medicine.

It was one of the best choices I ever made in my life. The world of plants has opened me up to a profound world of healing And it was only a little while ago I learned from one of my older cousins, a grandson of Dr. HW Partlow, that our ancestor HW had two offices in Olympia's Security Building: one was his treatment room and the other was stuffed full of HW's favorite healing herbs.

So it all comes around, full circle.

My formal herbal training
Clinical Herbalist Certification Program
                       KP Khalsa   1998-1999
Clinical Herbalist Apprenticeship

KP Khalsa   1999
International Certification Course in Aromatherapy
Kurt Schnaubelt   2000
East-West Herb Course
Michael & Leslie Tierra 2001
Therapeutic Herbalism Correspondence Course
David Hoffman   2002
Spirit of the Plants (Plant Spirit Medicine)
Joyce Netishen   2001-2002
Foundations in Herbal Medicine
Dr. Tierona LowDog 2002
Pacific School of Herbal Medicine
Adam Seller   2002
The Science & Art of Herbalism
Rosemary Gladstar   2004
California School of Traditional Hispanic Herbalism
Charles Garcia   2005

I became a professional member of the American Herbalist Guild in 2001.

Other formal plant & botany studies
Botany 112, South Puget Sound Community College
Laine McLaughlin   2002
Wetland Plants of the Northwest, UW Extension
Sarah Cooke   2004

Other important teachers, many of whom I know from their books
Juliette de Bairacli Levy
Michael Moore   Medicinal Plants of the Pacific West
Christopher Hobbs   Medicinal Mushrooms
Nancy Phillips   The Herbalist's Way
David Winston   Adaptogens
Matthew Woods   The Earthwise Herbal
Rosita Arvigo   Rainforest Remedies

I owe a special thanks to two of my earliest herbal teachers: Elise Krohn and Joyce Netishen who have walked the beauty way of plants as long as I have known them and have been very generous in sharing their knowledge with me and others. I am very grateful to have had the opportunity to walk alongside them.

www.ingramcontent.com/pod-product-compliance
Lightning Source LLC
Chambersburg PA
CBHW070253290526
45789CB00004B/1839